This Virus...

We Might Be Worried, But We Don't Need To Be.

A Book to Help Kids Deal with the Worries of Coronavirus

Written by Simone Hubble from happy hubble

We have a virus making its way around the world. **_We might be worried, but we don't need to be._** We might see adults getting worried and buying way too many things at the shops. Some are even overfilling their trolleys!

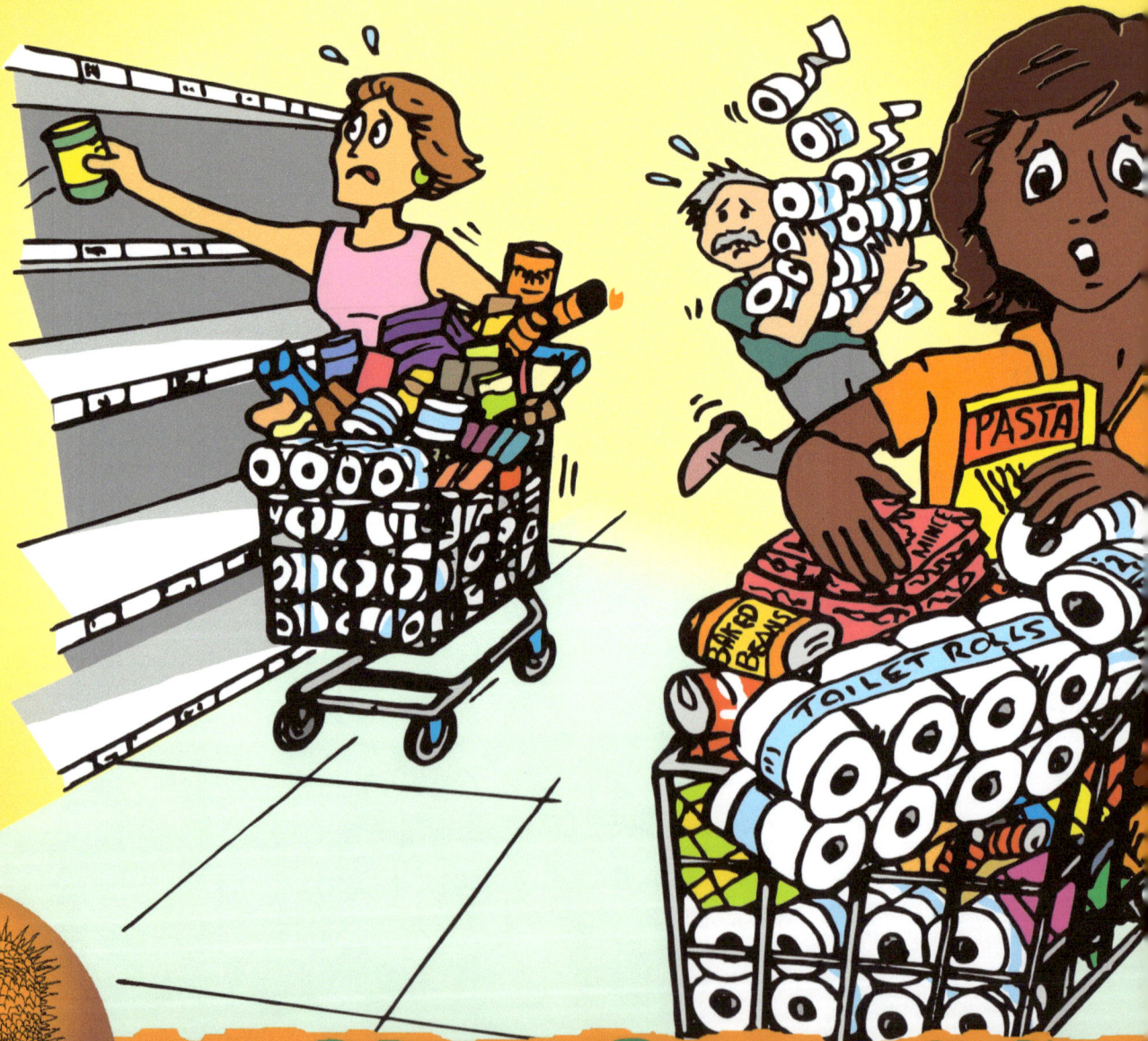

It makes them feel more prepared by having all the supplies they need at home for a very long time.

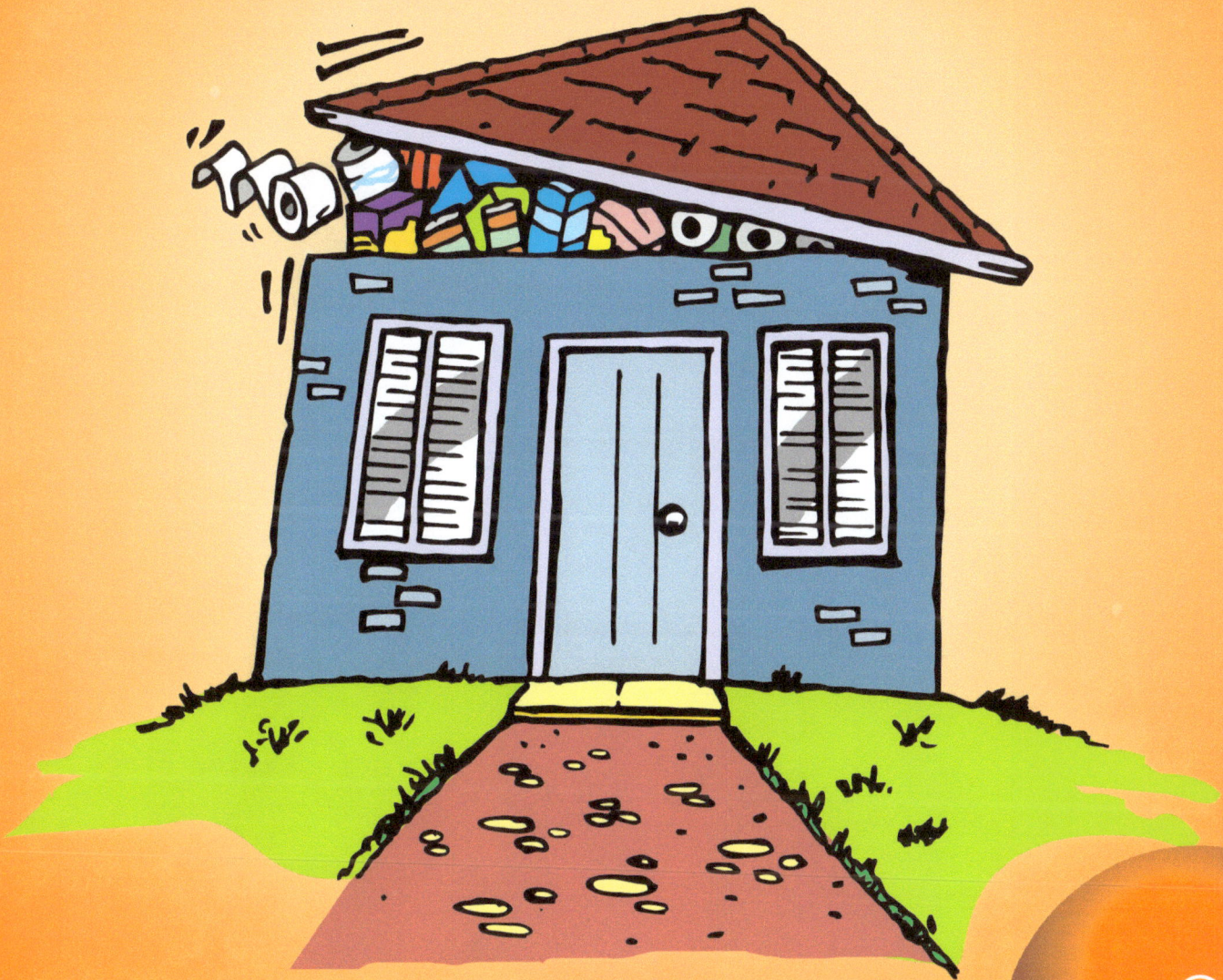

We might see adults yelling at each other or hurting each other, fighting over supplies at the shops.
There is plenty of food and supplies for everyone if we all work together.

We might be worried, but we don't need to be.

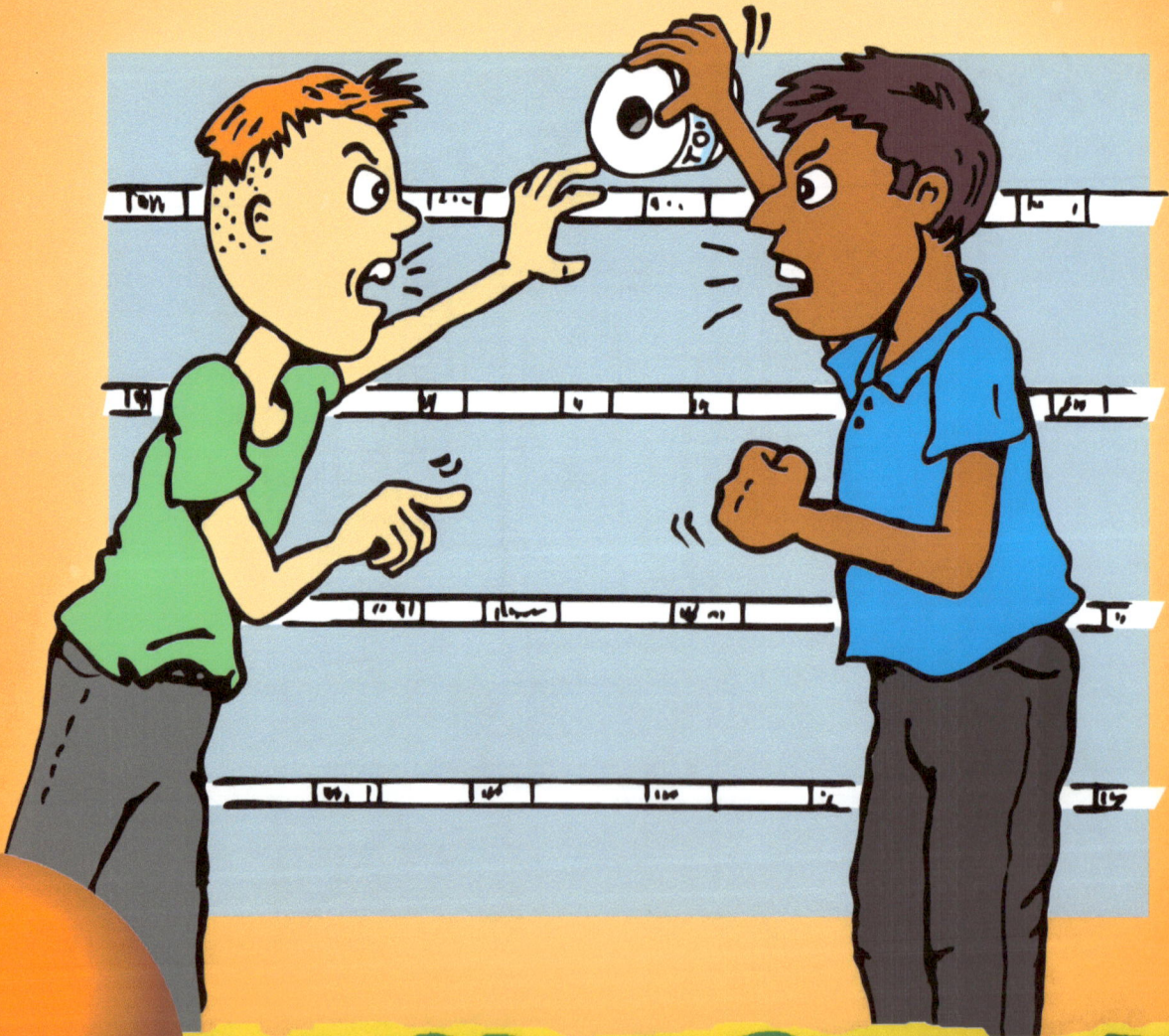

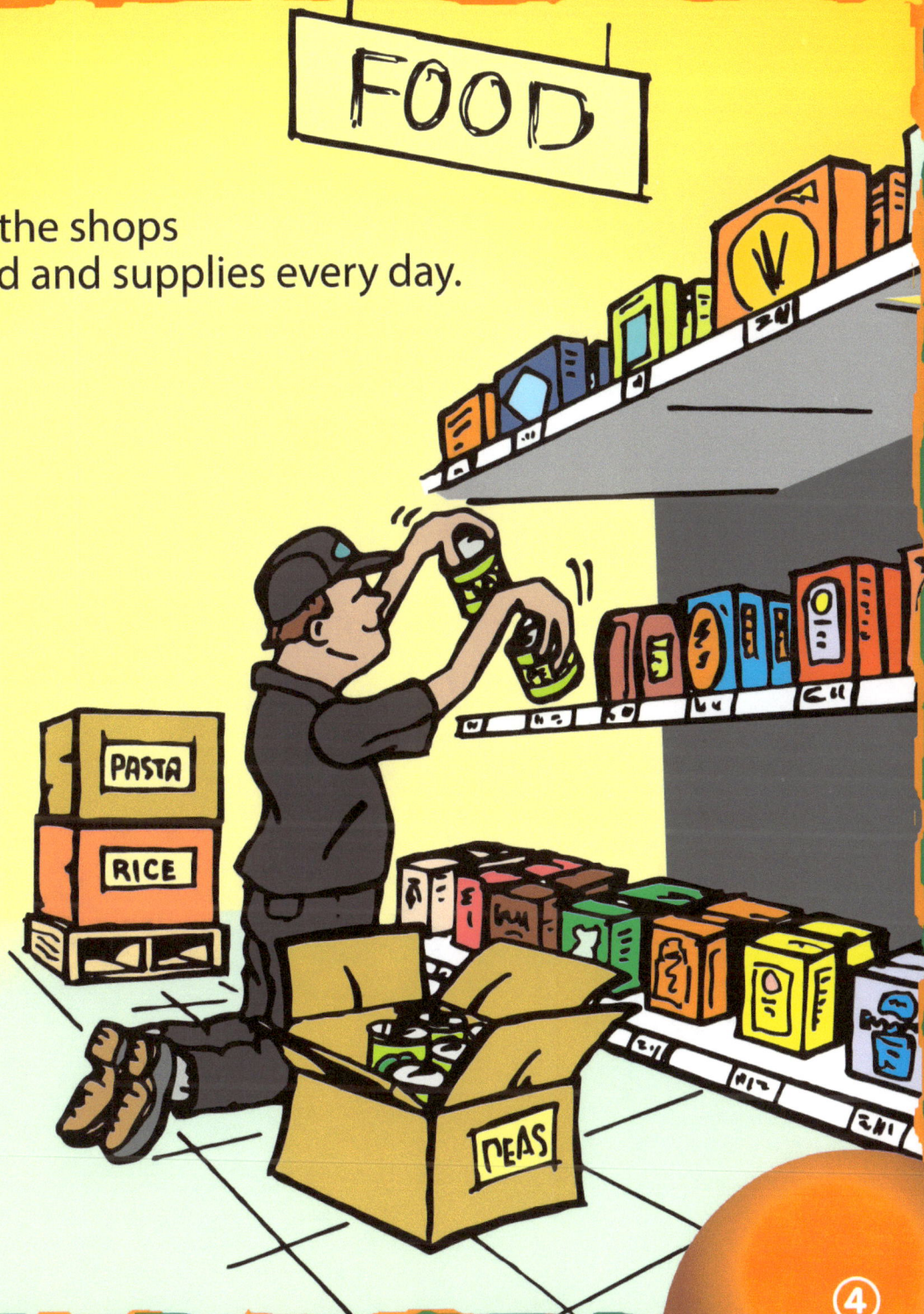

The workers at the shops
bring more food and supplies every day.

FOOD

PASTA

RICE

PEAS

We might be worried, but we don't need to be.

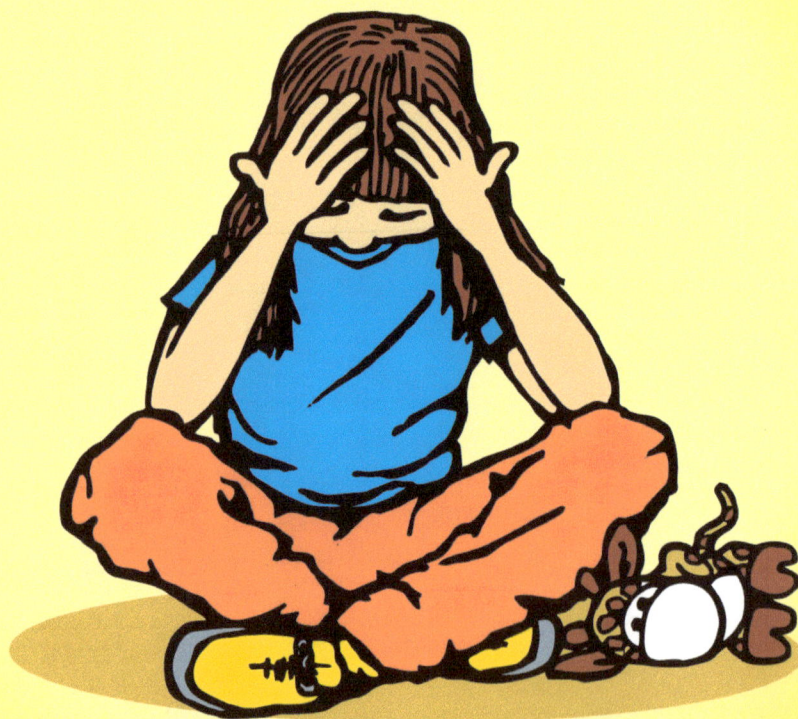

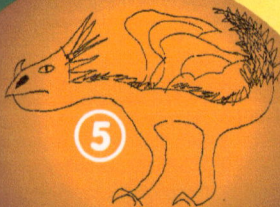

My friend
became ill

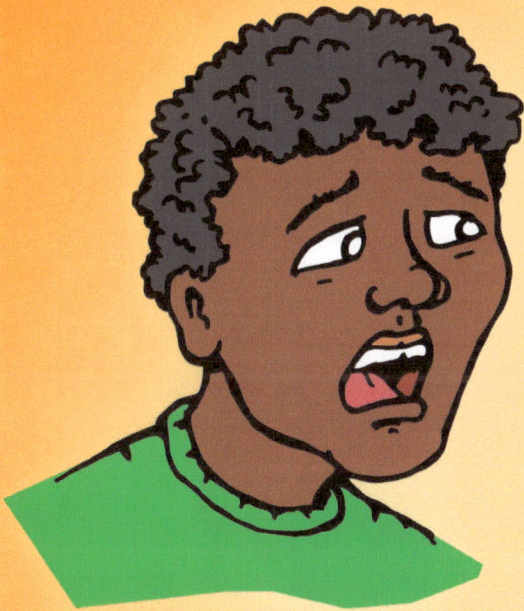

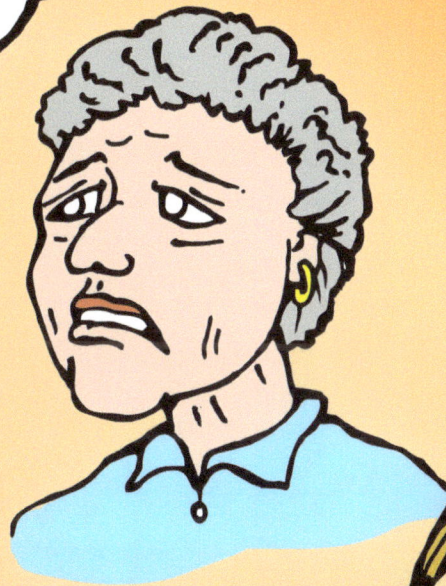

You may hear people
talking about getting sick.

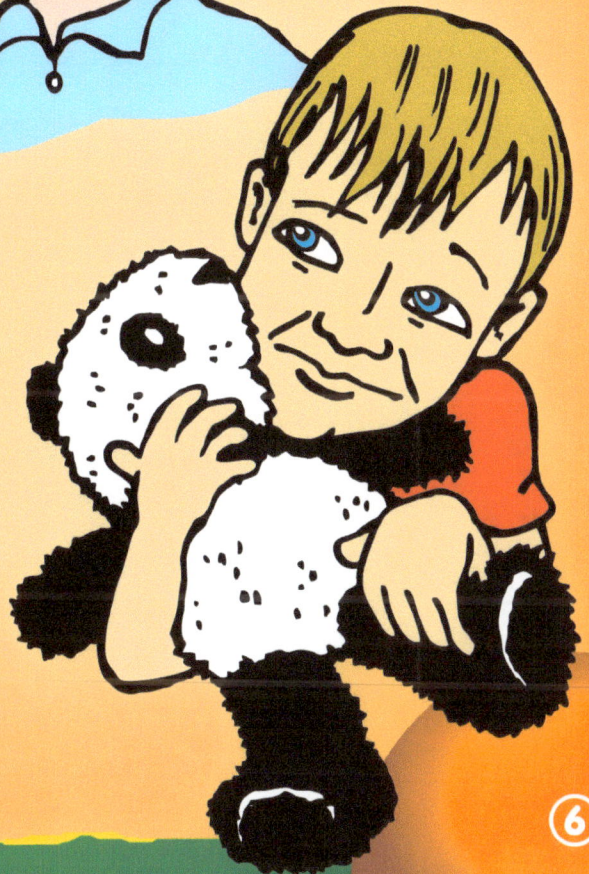

6

We might be worried, but we don't need to be.

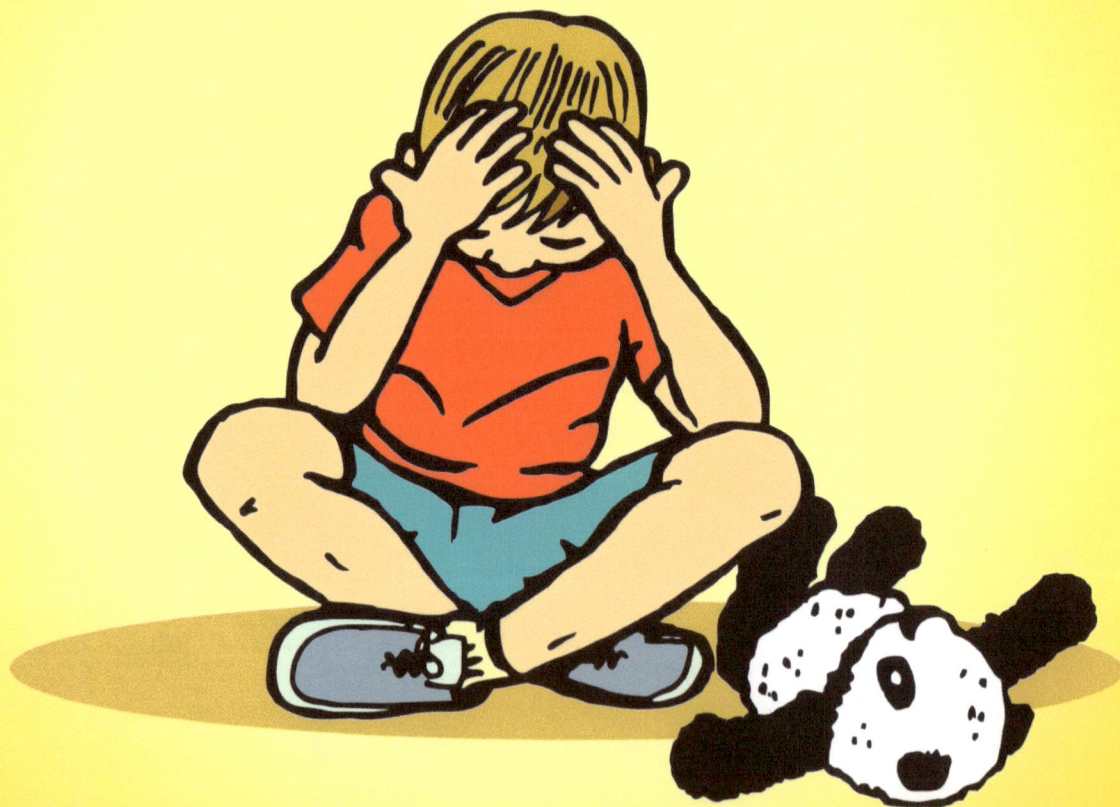

You may see scary things on the TV or a device.
Pictures of people in masks and
people in hospital beds.
Pictures of people crying or hurt.
You may even see world leaders
arguing with each other.
You might hear them
talk about the number of
sick people in the world
and how many have died.

**We might be worried,
but we don't need to be.**

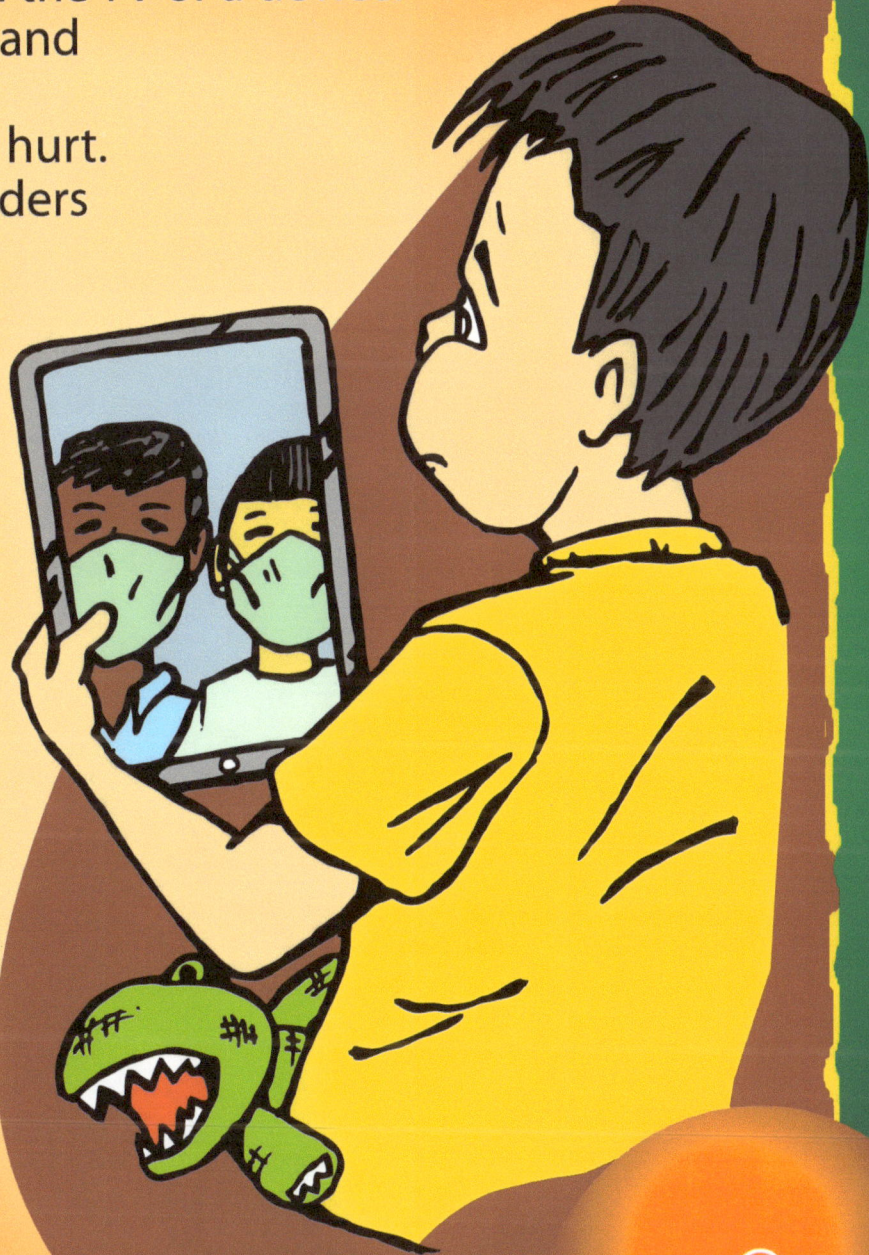

Sicknesses are not usually dangerous.
Some people may get sick but
most people will get better.

We might be worried, but we don't need to be.

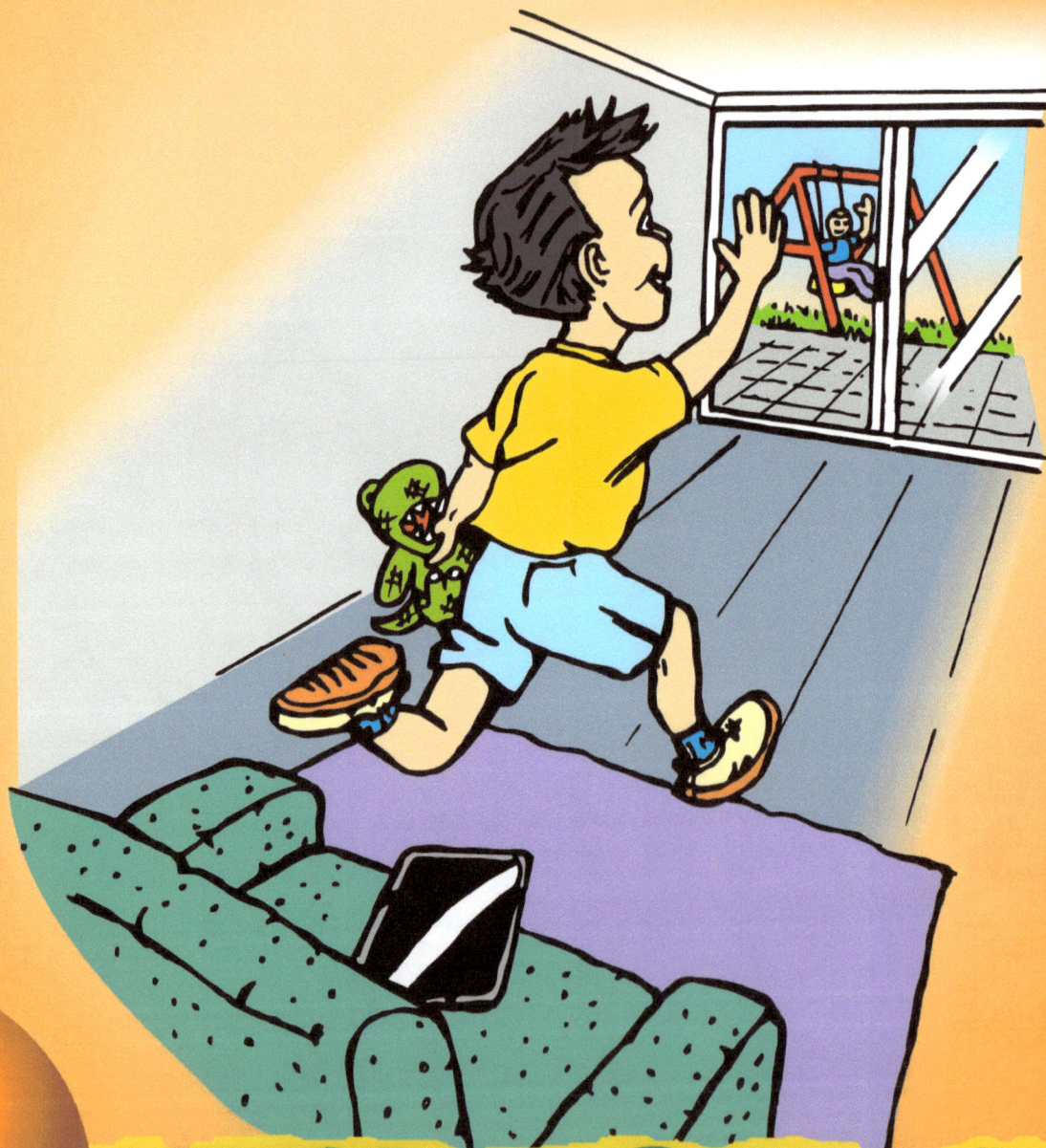

It just <u>sounds</u> scary at the moment.

Worried people can cause more worry. Here's what you can do...

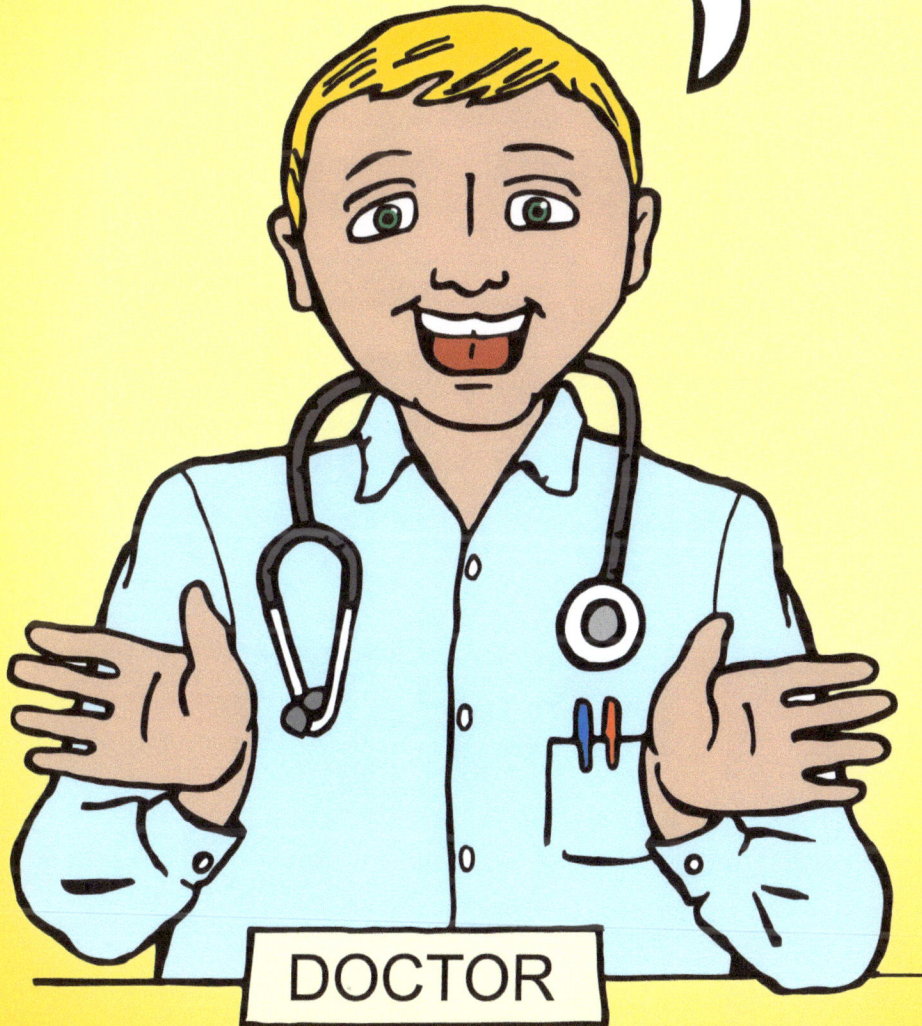

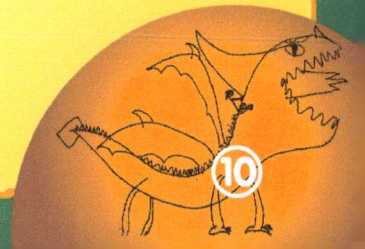

DOCTOR

10

Ask your parent, teacher or carer what is happening and they should give you the right answers. Sometimes the news on TV or a device can make things sound worse than it is.

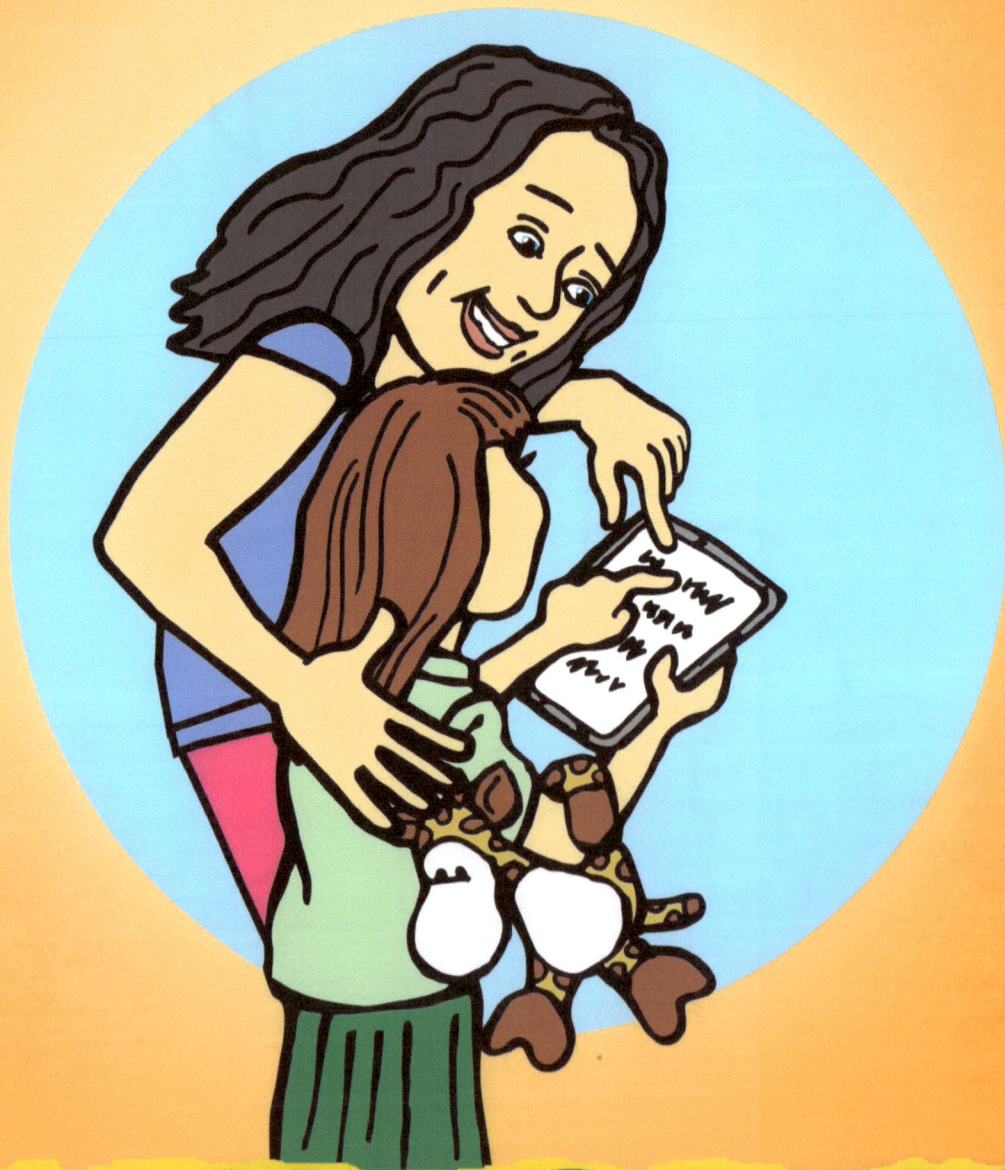

Just like any cough or cold, don't share your germs with anyone.
Use a tissue to cover your mouth when you cough,
or sneeze into your upper sleeve. After you blow your nose,
put the tissue in the bin.

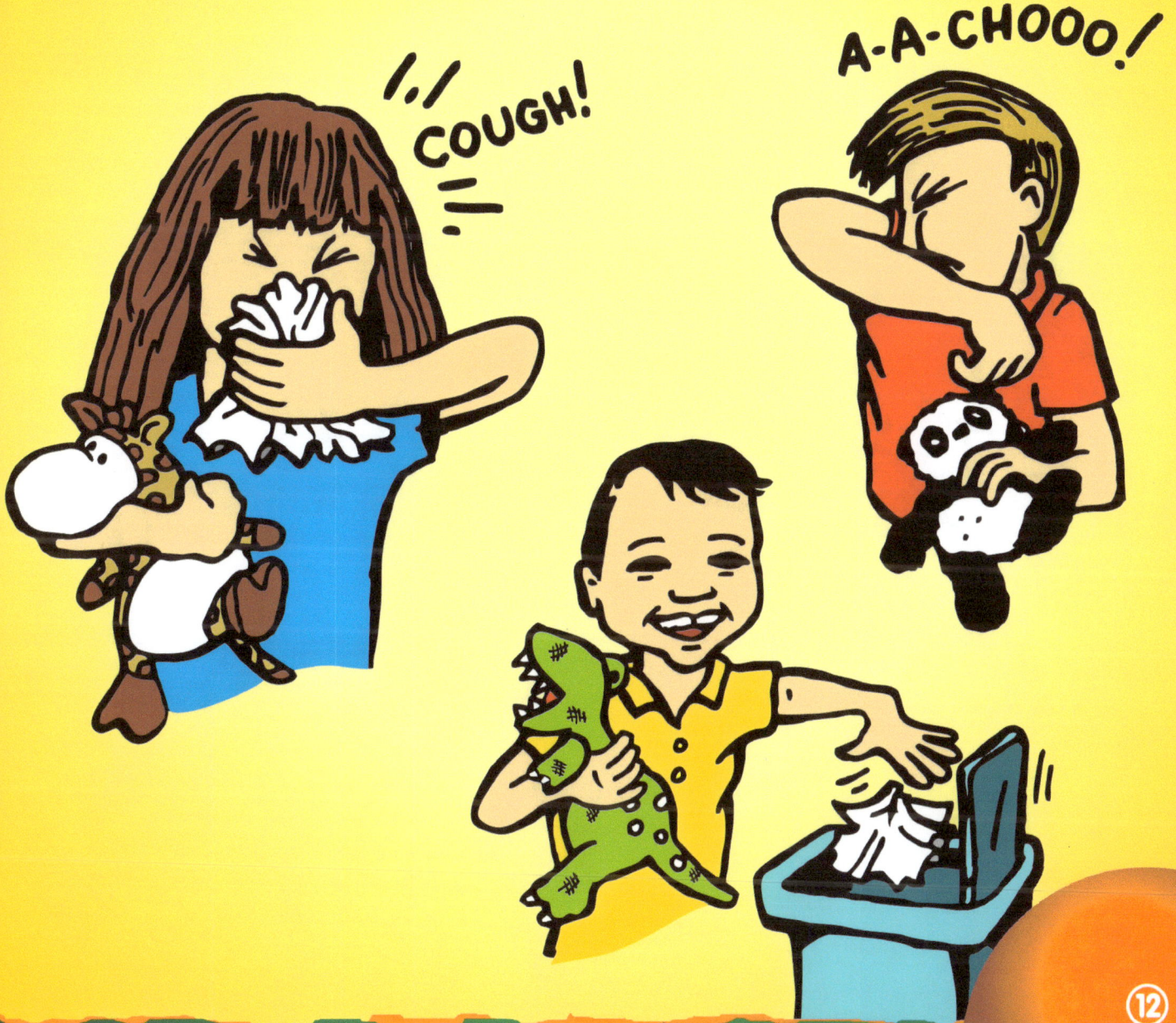

Wash your hands whenever they are dirty,
before you eat and after blowing your nose
or coughing.
If you can't get to soap and water,
use hand sanitiser.

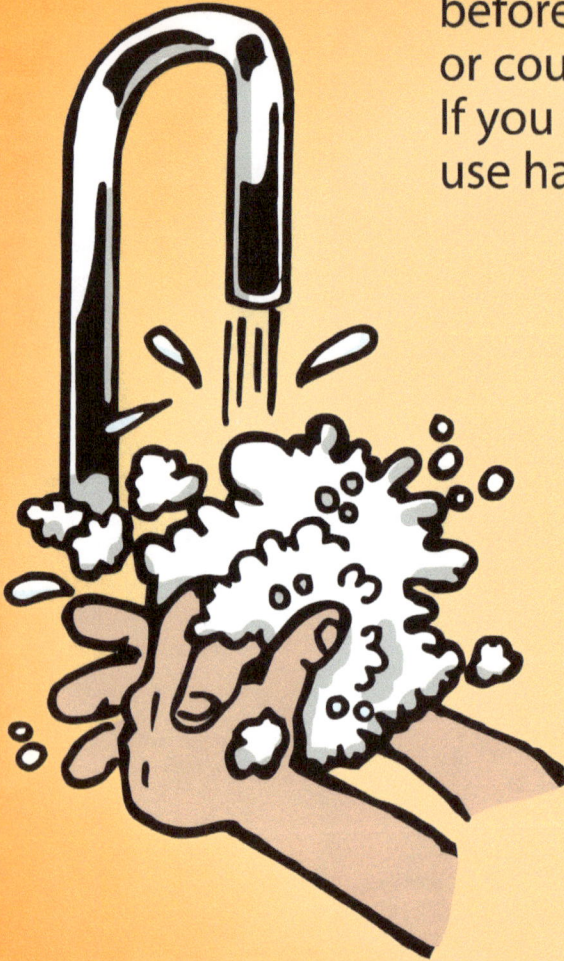

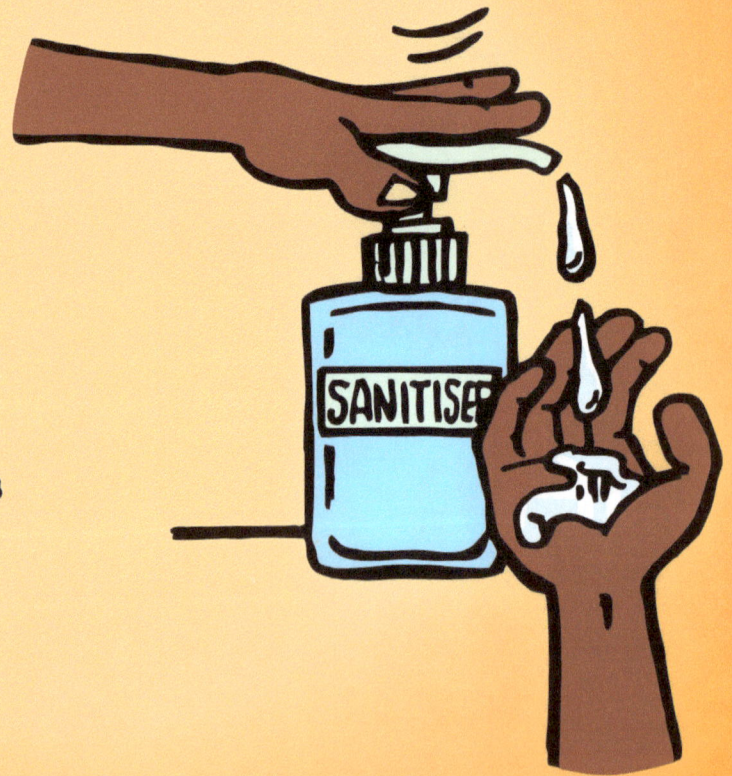

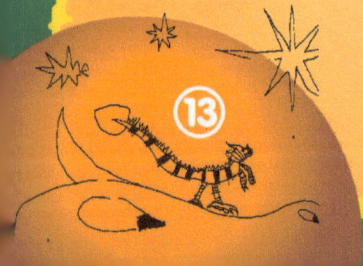

SANITISER

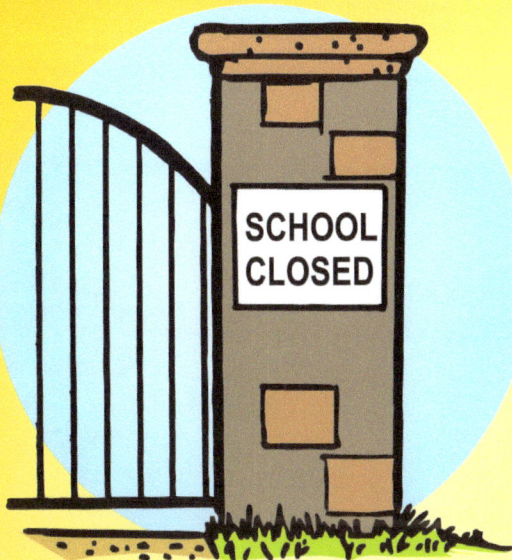

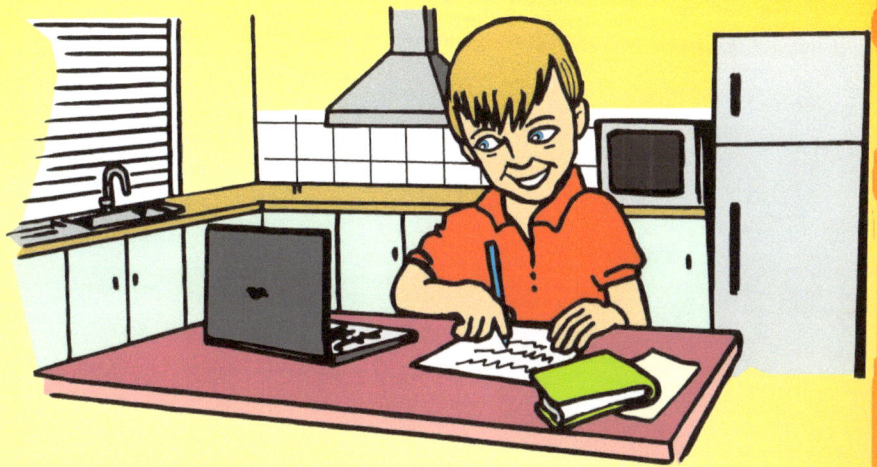

My school may close but I can learn from home.

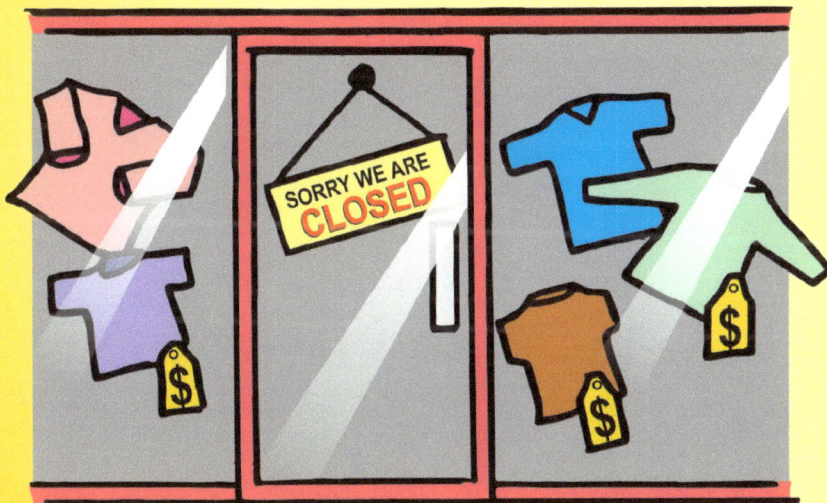

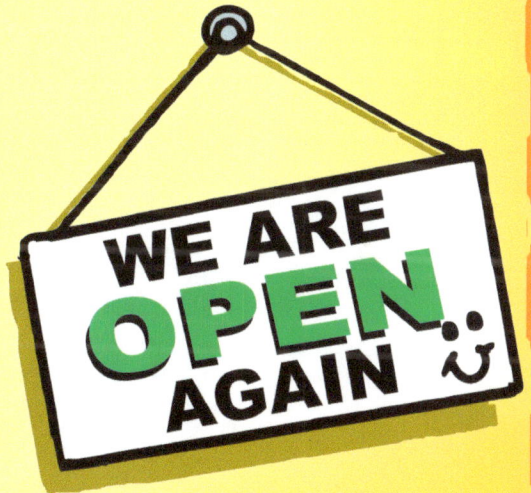

Some shops may close but everything will open again when all the people get better from this virus.

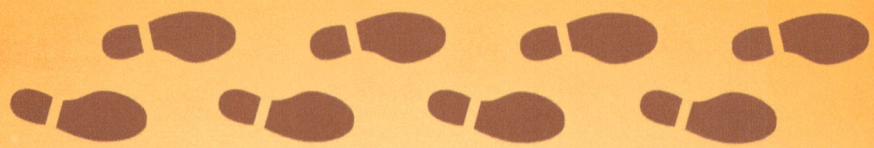

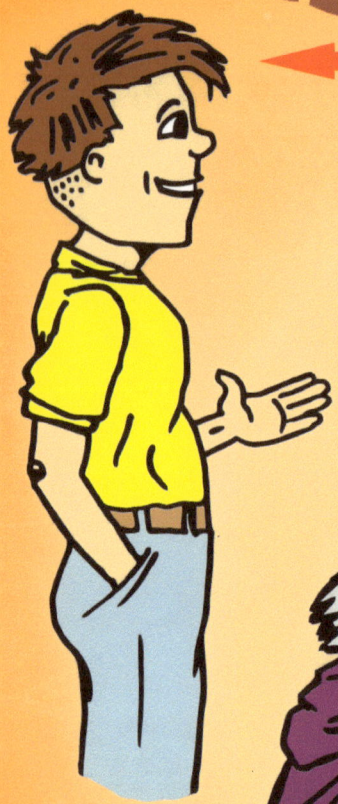

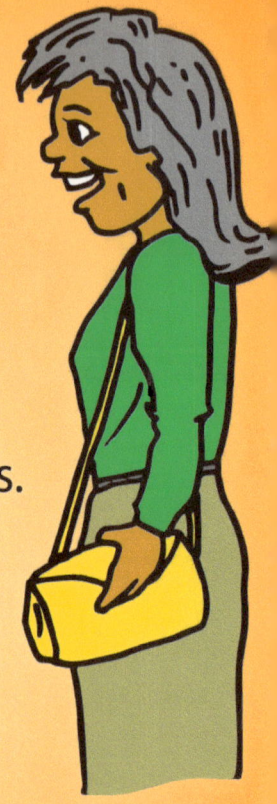

We need to stay home if we can, and if we do go out, stay a few steps away from people so we don't pass the virus around.

When we get home, we need to wash our hands for twenty seconds.

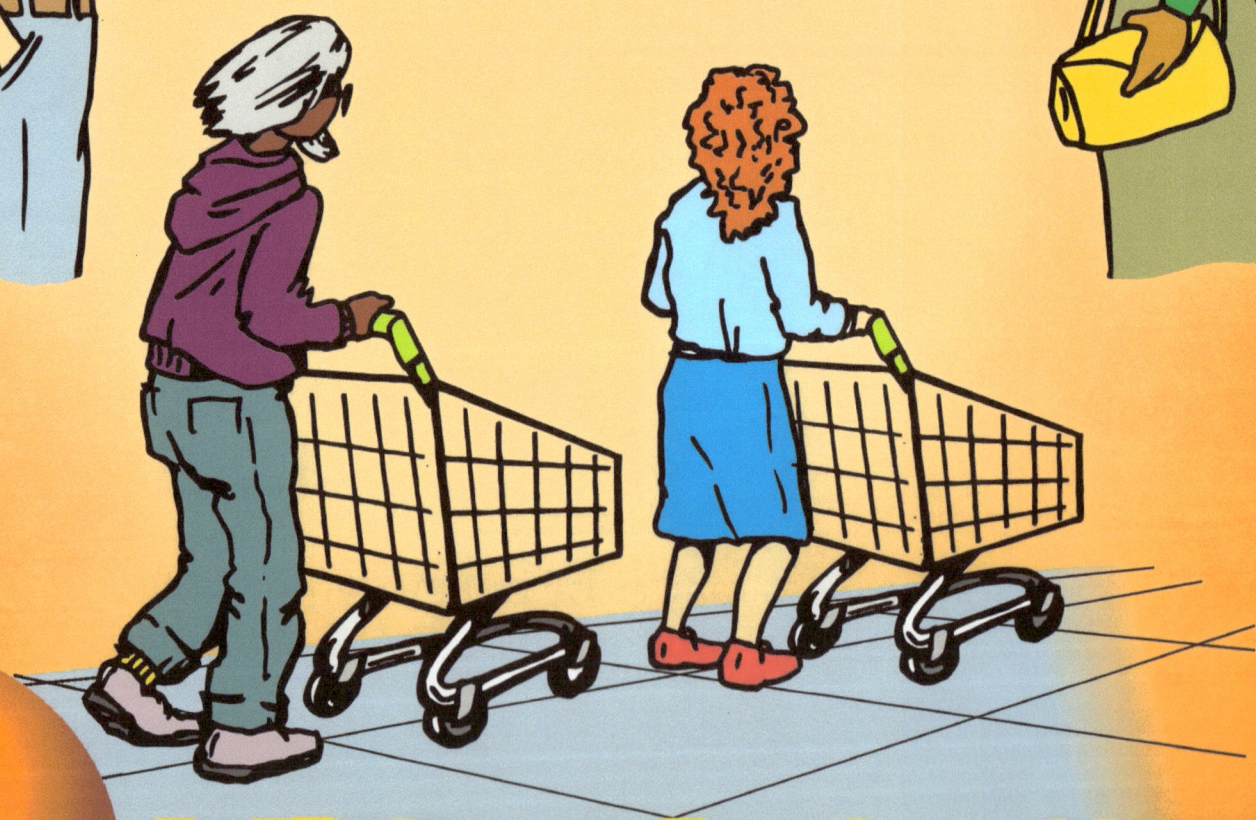

We can use our computer or device to have a video chat with our teacher, therapist, grandparents and friends.

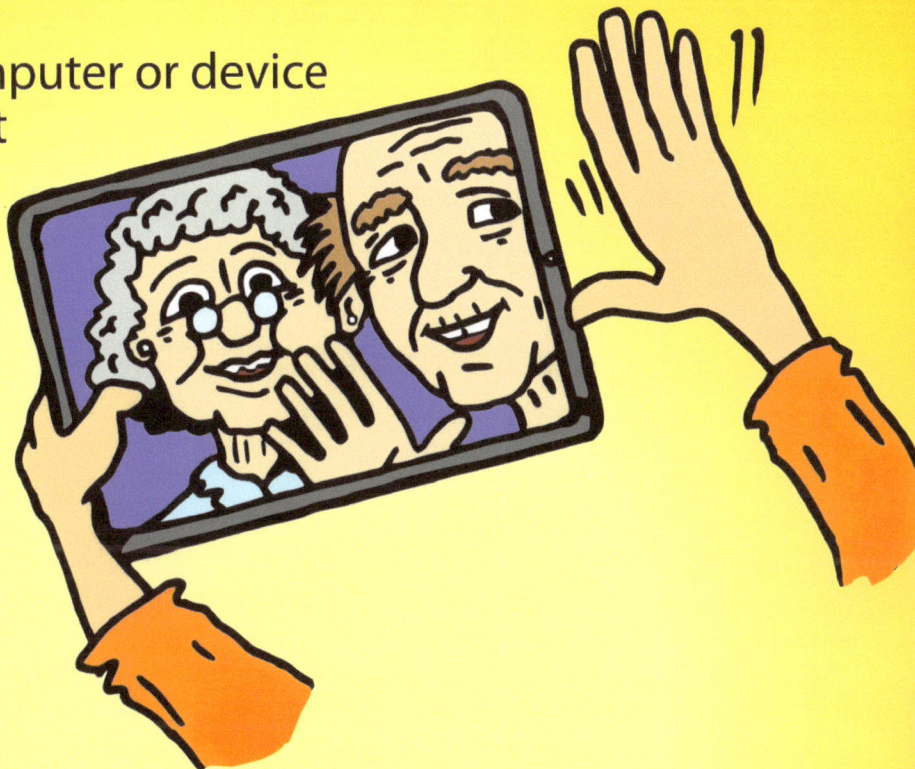

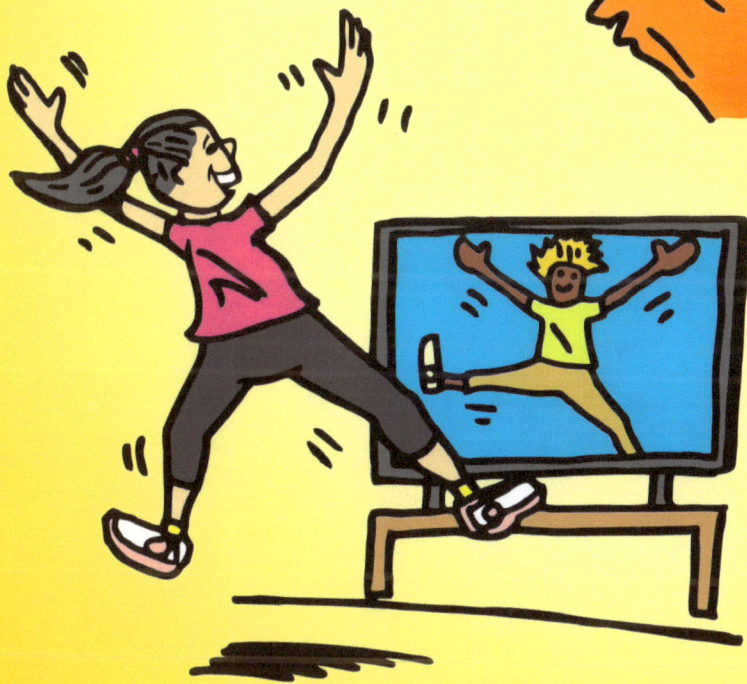

We can even use it to keep up with fun stuff like exercise classes, karate lessons and music lessons.
My mum is even doing Zumba classes in the living room!

You can't change what is happening with the virus, but you can change the way you think about it.
Remember, when you worry, it's best to talk to someone about how you feel.
Try taking slow breaths in and out, imagine something beautiful and peaceful.
Hugs with a special someone or something helps too!

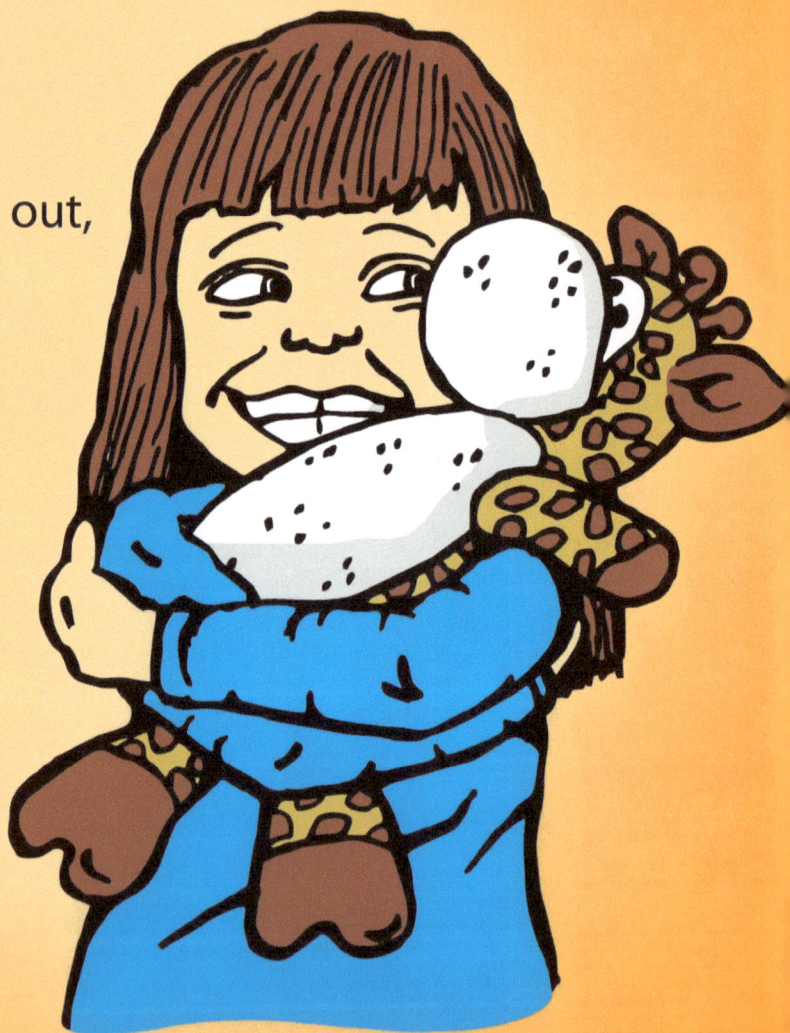

Stick to these few things
and you should be ok.
Remember scientists are
always working on a cure,
and importantly share this
advice and hopefully
the worry will be over soon.

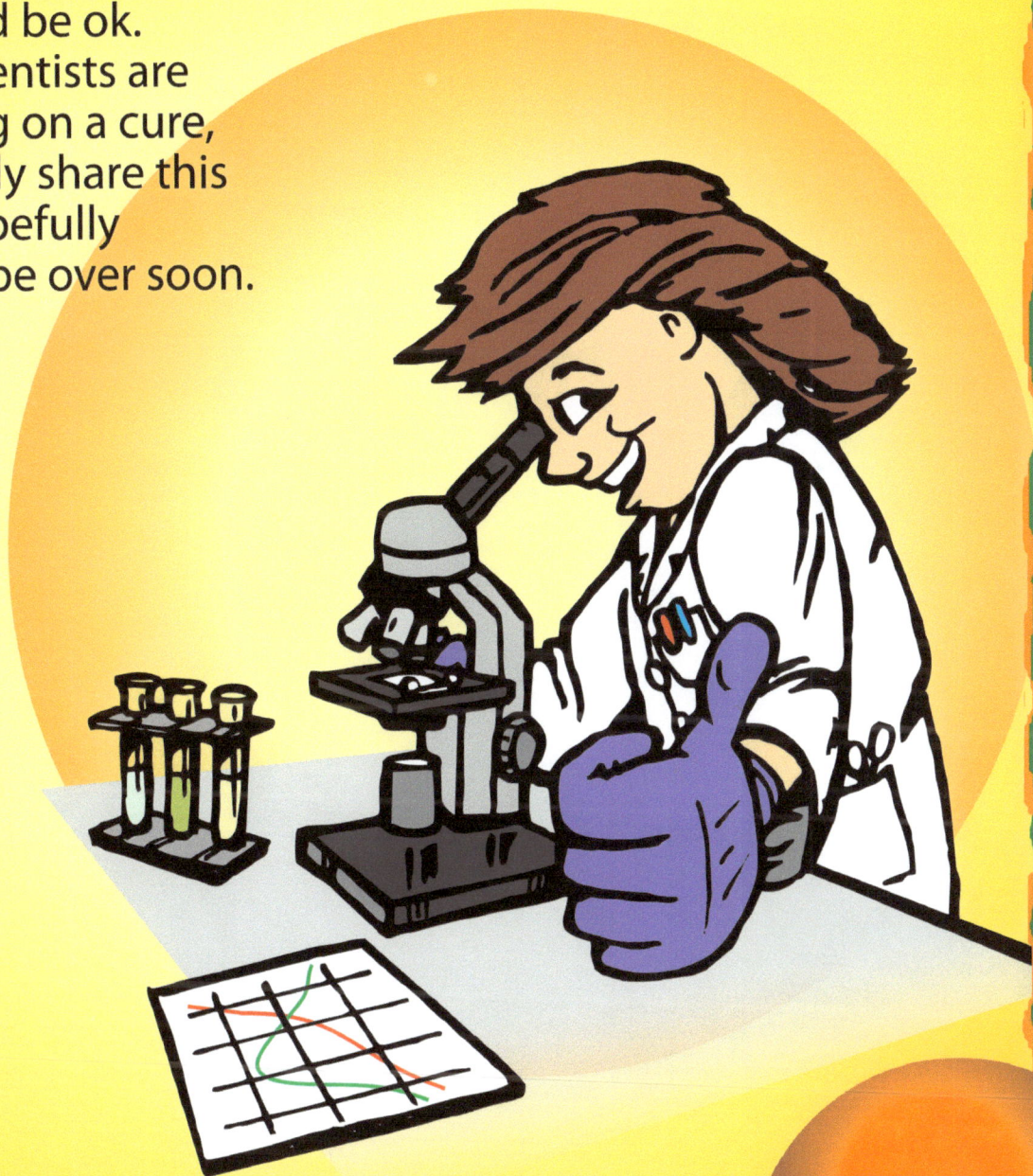

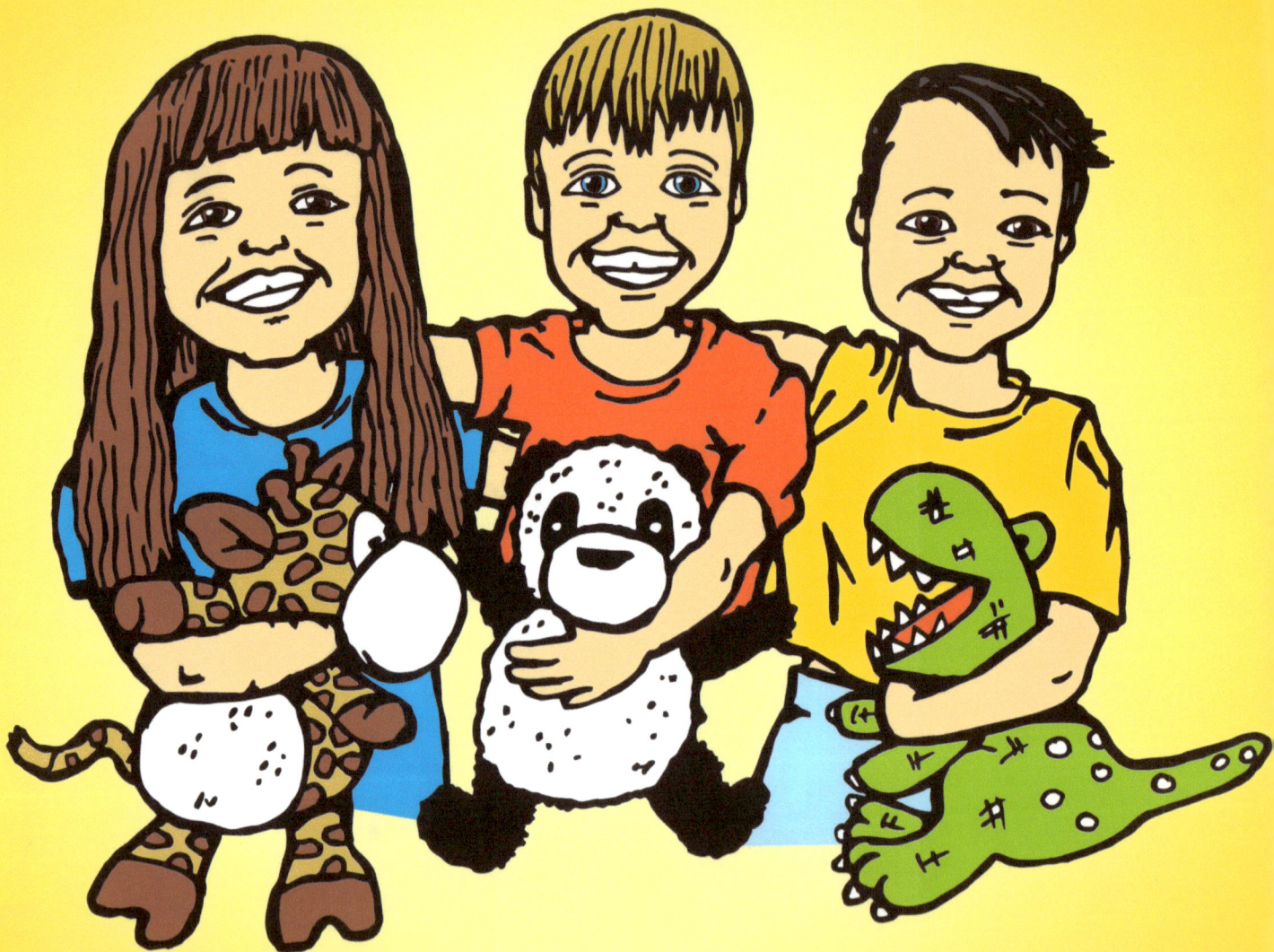

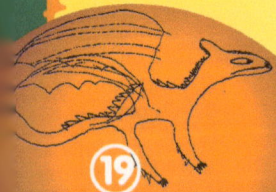

We might be worried, but we don't need to be.

About The Author

We are a young family who thought we had it all worked out.
We would have cute babies who would grow into happy,
easy-going children. We did have cute babies - three of them,
they did grow into happy children but they're not easy-going.
All three of our children are diagnosed with autism.

We love them to bits and we support them as best as we can,
but this support comes with so many challenges. They're not
easy, they need so much help and so many strategies to get
them through the simplest of everyday tasks. And they are all
so very different to each other. What works for one child
does not work for another. Without the right tools, I can soon
have three screaming children on my hands.

It's when we are given such an enormous and seemly
impossible task that we come up with fantastic strategies.
So, after looking for tools to help my kids, I decided to make
my own. My tools and ideas have interested our therapists
over the years. They have told me time and time again to
produce these tools for other parents. So I did and **'happy
hubble'** was born.

One of the popular tools to help our kids are "Social Stories",
these can help all children to visualise what is going to happen
and can help to lower their anxiety.

This is a life that found me. I was certainly not looking for it
and it has changed me forever. I live and breathe the needs
of our children. I've learnt how to look after them and how to
look after myself. Hopefully my knowledge will help others.

Simone Hubble

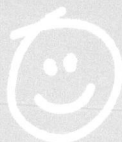

We might be worried, but we don't need to be.

www.ingramcontent.com/pod-product-compliance
Lightning Source LLC
Chambersburg PA
CBHW060846270326
41933CB00003B/208